THE
CBD OIL
SOLUTION

Learn How CBD Hemp Oil Might Just
Be The Answer For Pain Relief, Anxiety,
Diabetes and Other Health Issues!

Randolph Brennan

MEDICAL DISCLAIMER: The information contained in this book is intended for general information purposes only. You should always see your health care provider before administering any suggestions made in this book. Any application of the material set forth in the following pages is at your discretion and is your sole responsibility.

ERRORS

Please contact me if you find any errors.

My publisher and I have taken every effort to ensure the quality and correctness of this book. However, after going over the book draft time and again, we sometimes don't see the forest for the trees anymore.

If you notice any errors, I would really appreciate it if you could contact me directly before taking any other action. This allows me to quickly fix it.

Errors: errors@semsoli.com

REVIEWS

Reviews and feedback help improve this book and the author.

If you enjoy this book, I would greatly appreciate it if you were able to take a few moments to share your opinion and post a review online.

Table of Contents

Introduction

From online forums to the neighborhood coffee shop, it seems that everyone is talking about CBD (Cannabidiol) oil, the new wonder drug made from cannabis that, surprisingly, does not get you high. People claim that it has numerous health benefits and can cure dozens of diseases. Is CBD oil everything it claims to be?

In this book, author Randolph Brennan takes you on an in-depth journey to uncover everything you need to know about CBD oil. The author explores what CBD is, how it is produced, its differences from THC (Tetrahydrocannabinol) and how it affects your body. He also explores the major health benefits of CBD to help you know if CBD oil is right for you. He also highlights the main things you need to consider when buying CBD oil. In this book you will find a full breakdown on how to use CBD oil if it is your first time, and also read success stories of real life people who have achieved positive results with CBD oil. Finally, Randolph Brennan also highlights common myths and misconceptions about CBD to help you separate fact from fiction.

By the time you finish 'The CBD Oil Solution', you will have a clear understanding of how CBD oil can help you improve your quality of life and how to get started with CBD oil products.

Ready to learn about this new wonder drug that will change your life? Let's jump right in!

CHAPTER 1: What Is CBD Hemp Oil

In the last few years, there has been significant growth in the popularity of legal marijuana use, and other cannabis products, both for recreation and for their remarkable medicinal value.

With recent research showing that there are numerous medical benefits to be gained from the chemical compounds found in cannabis plants, there has been a surge in the number of people searching for cannabis products. The most popular of these products is CBD hemp oil. The popularity of CBD hemp oil stems from the fact that it is a natural remedy for numerous health problems. CBD has been shown to provide relief for all kinds of illnesses and conditions, from epilepsy and diabetes to anxiety and depression.

CBD hemp oil is a natural oil that has a high concentration of the chemical compound referred to as cannabidiol or CBD, which is found in cannabis plants. CBD oil is made by extracting cannabidiol from the hemp plant, and then mixing the cannabidiol with a carrier oil like hemp seed oil, olive oil, or coconut oil. It is important to note that while all cannabis plants contain CBD, CBD oil is extracted specifically from hemp plants, not marijuana. Hemp and marijuana are both cannabis plants, but they have one major difference. The hemp plant has a high concentration of CBD and a low concentration of THC (usually less than 0.3%), whereas marijuana plants are high in THC (which is why they get you high) and low in CBD. Extracting CBD from marijuana would lead to CBD oils with a high concentration of THC, the CBD oil made from hemp only contains trace amounts of THC.

What Is CBD?

Cannabis plants contain naturally occurring chemical compounds known as cannabinoids. Cannabinoids are a group of chemical compounds that bind with and act on cannabinoid receptors within the body's central regulatory system. There are three classes of cannabinoids: endocannabinoids (those produced naturally by the body), phytocannabinoids (those that occur naturally in plants) and synthetic cannabinoids (artificially manufactured). The cannabis plant contains about 113 phytocannabinoids. CBD is one of these cannabinoids. It is the second most prevalent cannabinoid in the cannabis plant, accounting for up to 40% of extracts from the plant. CBD is usually found within the flowers and the buds of hemp and marijuana plants. With all of this marijuana talk, know that CBD is a non-psychoactive compound. This means that it does not alter a person's mental state or affect a person's cognitive abilities. In addition, CBD does not have any addictive effects, it is very safe to use. CBD has a number of therapeutic properties, which explains its popular use as a relief for multiple ailments. Specifically, CBD is said to be anti-inflammatory, antioxidant, anticonvulsant, analgesic, antitumoral, antipsychotic, anti-nausea and anti-emetic, and anxiolytic. It is also an immune-modulator and a neuroprotector, and there's evidence that it helps to reduce the craving for alcohol, cocaine, heroin and even tobacco.

What Is The Difference Between CBD And THC?

There is a lot of public confusion about the difference between CBD (Cannabidiol) and THC (tetrahydrocannabinol). As a matter of fact, until recently, even the scientific community thought that CBD and THC were one and the same. The confusion stems from the fact that the two are the most prevalent cannabinoids found in the cannabis plant and they are very similar at the molecular level. In addition, both of them have an effect on the central nervous system.

The two cannabinoids actually have the same molecular makeup. Both CBD and THC contain 2 oxygen atoms, 21 carbon atoms and 30 hydrogen atoms. Despite these similarities, there is one key difference between CBD and THC. The arrangement of these atoms is not the same. It is because of this difference in atomic arrangement, CBD and THC have different effects on the body. THC binds with the Cannabinoid 1 (CB1) receptors in the brain, causing a sense of euphoria. Because of this, THC is termed as a psychoactive compound which means that it alters the state of the mind. The 'high' people experience after smoking marijuana is caused by the THC in marijuana. CBD, on the other hand, does not bind with CB1 receptors and is therefore non-psychoactive. You won't get high after using CBD products. Actually, CBD has been shown to be antagonistic to the psychotic effects of marijuana. This means that CBD can be used to counter the anxiety and cognitive impairment that is associated with marijuana. So while CBD is great for many health issues, it cannot be used for recreational purposes.

Due to its mind-altering effects, products containing THC are classified as psychotropic drugs and are strictly controlled by federal authorities across the world. CBD, on the other hand, does not have any psychotropic effects, therefore CBD products are legal in many parts of the world and are considered safe for human use. The fact that CBD products are legal and safe to use, in addition to the fact that they do not get people high, has hugely contributed to the growing popularity and social acceptability of CBD oils. You can gain their potential health benefits without the risk of jail time or the euphoric sensations (after all you don't necessarily want your mind altered on a normal day) associated with marijuana.

How Does CBD Work?

How does CBD affect your body? What happens when you use CBD products? When CBD gets into your body, it goes directly to the endocannabinoid system, which contains cannabinoid receptors. These receptors are found in different parts of your body: the brain, the skin, the immune cells, glands, different organs, connective tissue and so on. The endocannabinoid system is a physiological system within the body whose role is to establish and maintain homeostasis, which is crucial for human health. The endocannabinoid system releases endocannabinoids into your body, which then activate the cannabinoid receptors. Once these receptors are activated, they respond by regulating the functions of various systems in the body such as the digestive, reproductive, immune, endocrine, and the nervous systems, as well as the heart. The endocannabinoid system is also responsible for regulating other processes such as sleep, memory, appetite, mood, pain sensation, pleasure and reward, and so on. The aim is to ensure that your body is in a state of hemostasis, or optimal balance, at all times. This makes the endocannabinoid system very crucial in the establishment and maintenance of health within the body.

There are three types of cannabinoids – those produced by the body, those found in plants and artificially manufactured cannabinoids. When CBD enters your body, it activates the cannabinoid receptors just like the cannabinoids produced by your endocannabinoid system. Unlike some other cannabinoids like THC, CBD does not bind with the cannabinoid receptors. Instead, CBD inhibits some other cannabinoids from binding with the cannabinoid receptors, thus limiting the function of these other cannabinoids. This explains why CBD reduces the effects of THC in the body.

CBD also interacts with other receptors in the body, such as the nuclear receptors, serotonin receptors, orphan receptors, dopamine receptors, and vanilloid receptors. CBD also delays the reuptake of endogenous neurotransmitters. Since CBD positively interacts with the endocannabinoid system as well as other receptors that are responsible for maintaining health within the body, CBD products have such significant effects on health and wellness.

Chapter Summary

- There is increasing popularity in the use of cannabis products, and CBD oil in particular, as a natural remedy for different kinds of ailments.
- CBD hemp oil is a natural oil that has a high concentration of the chemical compound referred to as cannabidiol or CBD, which is found in cannabis plants.
- CBD oil is extracted specifically from hemp plants, not marijuana, since hemp plants have a lower concentration of THC.

- CBD or cannabidiol is one of the two important cannabinoids that occur naturally in cannabis plants.
- CBD is a non-psychoactive compound, which means that it does not alter a person's mental state or affect a person's cognitive abilities.
- CBD has a number of therapeutic properties, which explains its popular use as a relief for multiple ailments.
- CBD and THC have similar molecular structures but their atoms are arranged differently, which is why they have such different uses.
- THC is a psychoactive compound whereas CBD is non-psychoactive. CBD actually counters the effects of THC.
- THC products are strictly controlled by federal governments but CBD products are legal in many parts of the world and safe for human use.
- CBD works in the body by interacting with the endocannabinoid system, which is responsible for maintaining homeostasis within the body.

In the next chapter, you are going to learn about the health benefits of CBD hemp oil.

Chapter Two: Health Benefits Of CBD Hemp Oil

Despite the seemingly recent interest in the use of cannabis for health and wellness purposes, the idea that cannabis has health benefits is not a new one. In ancient China, hemp was commonly cultivated by farmers because of its many uses. Hemp's high-protein seeds were harvested for food while its fiber was used to make clothes and rope. Ancient Chinese physicians also used it for pain relief and to treat ailments such as malaria, rheumatism, gout and poor memory. Unfortunately, the use of cannabis for medicinal purposes declined after cannabis was classified as a schedule one drug and became a highly controlled substance. However, the use of cannabis as a natural remedy has started making a comeback.

A slowly growing body of research shows that the ancient physicians were actually onto something. Due to the status of cannabis as an illegal substance, the research on the health benefits of CBD oil is still in a nascent stage. Much of the research has also been based on animal studies. Although more studies and research are definitely needed to identify all the health benefits of CBD oil, several benefits have already been identified.

These include:

- Reduction Of Seizures In Epileptic Patients
- Anti-Inflammation And Pain Relief
- Anxiety And Mood Enhancement
- Lower Risk Of Cardiovascular Problems
- Helps With Management Of Diabetes
- Slows Progression Of Alzheimer's Disease
- Helps Combat Cancer
- Weight Loss
- Stronger Bones
- Helps With Smoking And Drug Withdrawal
- Better Sleep
- Treatment For Skin Conditions

Let's take a closer look at each of them.

Reduction Of Seizures In Epileptic Patients

CBD has properties that can help reduce seizures, especially in children who are resistant to conventional drugs. In one study carried out in Israel, children and adolescents diagnosed with intractable epilepsy were treated with a regimen of CBD-enriched medical cannabis. The study found that this treatment reduced the frequency of seizures by more than 50% among 52% of the patients. After research about the safety and effectiveness of CBD oil in reducing epileptic seizures, the US Food and Drug Administration (FDA) recently gave their approval for the use of Epidiolex, a CBD based prescription drug, as a treatment for two rare forms of epilepsy – Dravet Syndrome (DS) and Lennox-Gastaut Syndrome (LGS). These two types of seizures, which occur in children, have been shown to be resistant to other types of medication.

Anti-Inflammation And Pain Relief

CBD oils are great for relieving pain and stiffness. Since CBD oil is natural, it is a good alternative to prescription or over-the-counter pain relief drugs. It is also a good alternative for those dealing with chronic pain since it does not cause dependence and tolerance. Opioids, which are conventionally used to deal with chronic pain, are known to cause severe dependency issues. In patients with chronic pain, greater doses of opioids are needed over time due to increased tolerance. These are not concerns with CBD.

Several studies have been carried out to establish the effectiveness of CBD in pain relief. A study conducted by various universities in the United States and published in the *Journal of Experimental Medicine* found a link between CBD and reduced pain and inflammation in rats and mice. According to this study, CBD relieves pain by altering the response of pain receptors to stimuli. Another review of existing research by professors from the Faculty of Health and Life Sciences at the Pompeu Fabra University in Spain came to the conclusion that CBD may be an effective treatment for people suffering from Osteoarthritis. This view has been further reinforced by other studies conducted in the last few years.

While many of these studies have only been conducted on animals, there have been a few clinical trials. Even though the human trials have yet to provide conclusive results, a number of people suffering from inflammation-related diseases like arthritis claimed to have experienced a reduction in some of their symptoms after using CBD products.

Anxiety And Mood Enhancement

Use of CBD oil is often associated with a significant improvement in mood, a reduction in anxiety and a sense of pleasant calmness and bliss. The reduction of anxiety is attributed to the effect of CBD on 5-HT receptors. 5-HT receptors, also known as serotonin receptors, are responsible for regulating the release of neurotransmitters and hormones that influence processes such as mood, aggression, stress and anxiety. The anti-anxiety and mood enhancing properties of CBD are also linked to the effect of CBD on the limbic system in the human brain. CBD decreases activity in a section of the brain known as the amygdala which is responsible for the "fight or flight" response. Less activity in the amygdala leads to decreased panic, anxiety and stress.

The use of CBD as a remedy for stress and anxiety has a lot of academic support. In a 2011 study by researchers from the Department of Neuroscience at the University of Sao Paulo, a group of volunteers received either a dose of CBD or a placebo and were then subjected to a public speaking test. The study found that volunteers who received the placebo experienced higher levels of anxiety, discomfort and cognitive impairment during the public speaking test compared to those who received a dose of CBD. Yet another study by Brazilian researchers found that giving volunteers a dose of CBD lead to decreased levels of cortisol in the body. Cortisol is the body's stress hormone, with high levels of cortisol being associated with high levels of stress. Next time you are feeling stressed or anxious, take a dose of CBD oil. It is proven to help lift your spirits and improve your mood.

Lower Risk Of Cardiovascular Problems

Heart disease is becoming more common, especially in the United States. Actually, cardiovascular diseases are the leading cause of death in the United States, both among men and women. The truth is that no one is free from the risk of cardiovascular complications. They can happen to anyone and can be caused by any number of reasons. Fortunately, you can reduce your risk of suffering from cardiovascular disease by using CBD oil. Because it is a cannabinoid, there is no direct interaction between CBD and the cardiovascular system. However, the effects of CBD on the endocannabinoid system have an indirect effect on the cardiovascular system.

CBD reduces the risk of cardiovascular problems in three ways. First, CBD reduces inflammation. Sometimes, heart complications occur as a result of inflammation in the cardiovascular cells, which leads to the death of these cells. Inflammation of cardiovascular cells can be caused by many things. If left untreated, this inflammation can cause serious complications that might even result in death. The anti-inflammatory properties of CBD help prevent inflammation and the death of cardiovascular cells.

Secondly, use of CBD is sometimes associated with decreased blood pressure. This is often touted as a negative side effect of CBD. However, in the event of a heart attack, decreased blood pressure can literally save a person's life. CBD decreases blood pressure by widening blood vessels, which in turn allows more blood to flow. In a bid to establish the effects of CBD on blood pressure, one study gave healthy male volunteers a dose of CBD or a placebo and then took the volunteers through some tests designed to raise their blood pressure. The volunteers who received the dose of CBD had lower blood pressure, lower stroke volume, and a lower resting systolic pressure.

Finally, CBD is an anti-arrhythmic. A heart arrhythmia refers to a condition where your heart beats irregularly. This can either be too fast, too slow, too early, and so on. In most cases, heart arrhythmias do not lead to any problems. Sometimes, however, they can lead to complications, for example, when your heartbeat becomes exceptionally irregular. Fortunately, CBD can help restore your heartbeat to its regular rhythm. Studies conducted on rodents by researchers from the University of Strathclyde and the Robert Gordon University found that CBD is an effective treatment for heart arrhythmia even though they are not yet sure how CBD does this.

Helps With Management Of Diabetes

Diabetes has also become a very common illness, with millions of people in the world suffering from the disease. Complications resulting from diabetes are a major cause of premature death, with diabetics being three times more likely to suffer from heart complications and up to twelve times more likely to suffer from end-stage renal failure. For most people living with diabetes, the conventional treatment is a diet change and insulin. In recent years, huge numbers of people have been turning to CBD oil as an alternative treatment to help them manage the disease.

Diabetes is primarily a homeostasis problem, resulting from the inability of the body to regulate the levels of sugar in the blood. In type 1 diabetes, no insulin is produced by the pancreas, while in type 2 diabetes, the body does not respond to insulin as it should. Using CBD oil can help a person stabilize the levels of sugar in their blood. A 2013 paper published in the American Journal of Medicine said CBD can help lower insulin resistance by up to 17%, thereby helping reduce the effects of type 2 diabetes. CBD can also help reduce the effects of type 1 diabetes. Type 1 diabetes is usually caused by inflammation due to immune cells attacking the cells of the pancreas. CBD can help prevent this kind of inflammation and so it can help to protect the cells of the pancreas.

CBD oil has several other effects that make it easier to manage diabetes. Diabetes often causes blurry vision due to inflammation of the optic nerve. CBD oil helps prevent this inflammation of the optic nerve, preventing vision issues. CBD also prevents inflammation of other nerves within the body, a condition known as neuropathy, which is common with diabetics. Neuropathy results in nerve damage in the lower body, which is why some diabetics end up having their legs amputated. Also, remember how CBD deals with cardiovascular issues? CBD reduces blood pressure and keeps blood vessels open. This is very important for diabetics considering that they have an increased risk of heart complications. Finally, CBD acts as an antispasmodic agent, helping prevent gastrointestinal disorders and muscle cramping.

Due to these benefits, many diabetics are turning to CBD oil as one of the best natural remedies for the disease, with great results. While CBD oil does not actually cure the disease, it does make the disease more manageable. It's good to keep in mind that diabetes is quite a serious condition, if you have it, CBD oil therapy should only be used with supervision from a doctor or other health professional.

Slows Progression Of Alzheimer's Disease

Alzheimer's disease is a form of dementia. The disease causes deterioration of a person's memory and negatively affects their thoughts and behavior. This makes it difficult for the person to perform daily activities. In advanced stages, the disease makes life very difficult, both for the patient, caregiver and family members. So far, there is no known cure for Alzheimer's. However, CBD therapy has been shown to be effective in slowing down the progression of the disease.

Alzheimer's disease, as well as other neurodegenerative diseases are often worsened by inflammation of neural tissue. During the onset of the disease, inflammation occurs as the body's defense against the disease. However, this inflammation becomes uncontrollable, leading to chronic deterioration of neural tissue. Due to its anti-inflammatory properties, CBD can help stem the inflammation during the early stages, actually helping to slow down the disease.

Additionally, the inflammation of neural tissue leads to release of reactive oxygen in the brain. As more reactive oxygen is released into the brain, it causes the production of free radicals in the brain, which in turn react with proteins and fatty acids within cell membranes, causing breakdown of neurons and synapses within the brain. This causes loss of memory and other forms of brain deterioration. CBD oil can be used to counteract this effect. CBD oil is an antioxidant. It helps reduce the amount of reactive oxygen in the brain which can help prevent the loss of brain function that is associated with Alzheimer's.

A study conducted on mice in 2014 supports the claim that CBD oil can help slow the progression of Alzheimer's disease. The study found that CBD oil kept social recognition deficit at bay in the mice. Social recognition deficit is one of the common symptoms of Alzheimer's. The anti-inflammatory and antioxidant properties of CBD that make it effective in slowing the progress of Alzheimer's are also useful in reducing the progress of other neurodegenerative diseases, such as vascular dementia, Parkinson's disease, multiple sclerosis, and so on.

Helps Combat Cancer

CBD oil has also been shown to be effective in treating people with cancer. In a study to examine the effect of CBD on cancerous cells, scientists from the Complutense University in Madrid grew cancerous cells in a lab and then treated them with CBD. The team found that CBD killed the cancerous cells without causing any destruction to nearby healthy, non-cancerous cells. However, the team found that CBD was most effective against cancerous cells when combined with THC. CBD combats cancerous cells in two ways. First, it interferes with the cellular communication of cancerous cells. Second, CBD is capable of triggering apoptosis in cancerous cells. Apoptosis is the pre-programmed death of a cell.

The National Cancer Institute and the American Cancer Society officially recognize CBD oil as an effective treatment for slowing down the growth and spread of cancerous cells. CBD oil is specifically effective in combating the progression of prostate, lung, colon, and breast cancer. In addition to slowing down the growth and spread of cancer cells, CBD oil also effective in combating the nausea and vomiting that is associated with chemotherapy and relieving the pain caused by cancer.

Weight Loss

With the growing popularity of CBD oil, many athletes and fitness enthusiasts have also started using CBD oil as a natural solution for maintaining a healthy body weight. Normally, people associate cannabis products with increased appetite, especially when they hear marijuana smokers talking about the munchies. The increase in appetite experienced by marijuana users is a direct result of THC. The effect CBD has on appetite is the complete opposite. CBD suppresses appetite, which is a good thing for someone to lose weight.

In addition to suppressing appetite, CBD also boosts weight loss by increasing the activity within your mitochondria. Mitochondria are the powerhouses of the body. They are responsible for burning your calories and converting them into energy. Increased activity in the mitochondria means you will end up burning more calories and decrease the amount of fat in your body.

CBD oil also stimulates weight loss by accelerating a process known as fat browning. Fat browning is a process through which white fatty tissues are converted into brown fatty tissues. The body uses white fatty tissues to store calories but brown fatty tissues are ready to be converted into energy. By accelerating this process, CBD reduces the quantity of calories that get stored in the body as fat.

Stronger Bones

To maintain strong, healthy bones, the body naturally replaces old bone material with new and stronger bone material, in a process known as bone metabolism. This is a slow process, with about 10% of old material being replaced each year. Cannabinoids help facilitate this process. CBD in particular can help enhance the strength of your bones. CBD inhibits the release of an enzyme that is responsible for destroying bone building compounds.

Excess production of this enzyme limits the ability of the body to create new bone and cartilage cells, leading to diseases such as osteoarthritis and osteoporosis. By inhibiting the release of this enzyme, CBD encourages the formation of new bone cells, leading to stronger, healthier bones. CBD also speeds up the healing of fractures and reduces the risk of re-fractures.

Helps With Smoking And Drug Withdrawal

CBD is also effective in helping people quit their addiction to smoking and drug use. To test the effectiveness of CBD oil in minimizing the effects of withdrawal, a group of London based researchers conducted a short term study with a group of 24 smokers. Half the group of smokers were given inhalers containing CBD while the other half received inhalers with a placebo substance. The group was encouraged to use the inhalers whenever they felt like smoking. The study lasted a week. The results of the study, which were posted in the Addictive Behaviors journal, found that those who received the CBD inhaler reduced their cigarette consumption by about 40%. Those who received the placebo showed no difference in their cigarette consumption. While the results from the study are not conclusive, they do support the view that CBD can be used to treat nicotine addiction.

A review by a team of researchers from different universities in the United States and Canada published in the journal *Neurotherapeutics* came to the conclusion that CBD may be similarly effective in treating addiction to opioids. The team also noted that use of CBD is associated with a reduction in some of the symptoms of withdrawal from drug use, such as insomnia, pain, mood-related problems and anxiety.

Better Sleep

If you have sleeping problems, CBD oil can also help you sleep better. Most sleeping problems are caused by stress and anxiety, which makes it difficult for your brain to shut down. If your sleeping problems are caused by anxiety, using CBD oil can help calm down the anxiety, thus making it easier for you to fall asleep and even improve your quality of sleep. CBD regulates the amount of cortisol and adrenaline in your body, the two hormones responsible for stress and alertness. There is scientific backing for this claim. According to animal studies published in the journal *Current Psychiatry Reports* and the *Journal of Psychopharmacology*, CBD can help reduce insomnia and increase sleeping time.

Treatment For Skin Conditions

CBD oil has also been found to be very useful in the beauty industry. CBD oil is good for the skin for a number of reasons. First, it is good for the overall health of the skin since it contains some important nutrients, like vitamin E. CBD oil is also an effective treatment for acne. One of the causes of acne is the inflammation of the sebaceous glands in the skin. Inflammation of these glands leads to overproduction of sebum, leading to occurrence of acne. Due to its anti-inflammatory properties, CBD oil helps reduce the production of sebum, thus undoing the effects of acne. CBD oil can also be used as a treatment for other skin conditions such as eczema by triggering the apoptosis of abnormal skin cells.

Chapter Summary

- ☐ The idea that cannabis products have health benefits has been in existence for hundreds of years.
- ☐ A growing body of research confirms that some components of cannabis, such as CBD, can be used as remedies for some ailments.
- ☐ CBD has been approved by the FDA as an effective treatment for DS and LGS, two rare forms of epileptic seizures that are resistant to other types of medication.
- ☐ CBD can be used for pain relief and as a remedy for inflammation.
- ☐ Use of CBD oil can also help with anxiety and stress reduction and improvement of moods.
- ☐ Using CBD reduces your risk of developing cardiovascular problems and complications.
- ☐ CBD helps reduce the symptoms of both type 1 and type 2 diabetes and also helps diabetics in dealing with the pain associated with the disease.
- ☐ CBD can help slow the progress of Alzheimer's disease and other neurodegenerative diseases such

as vascular dementia, Parkinson's disease, and multiple sclerosis.

- CBD can help kill cancerous cells. It is also effective in combating the nausea and vomiting that is associated with chemotherapy and relieving the pain caused by cancer.
- Many athletes and fitness enthusiasts are also turning to CBD since it has been proven to be effective in helping people lose weight.
- CBD encourages the formation of new bone cells, leading to stronger, healthier bones.
- CBD has also been shown to be an effective treatment for addiction to nicotine and opioids. If you have sleeping problems, CBD oil can also help you sleep better.
- CBD also improves the health of your skin and is an effective treatment for skin conditions such as eczema and acne.

In the next chapter, you are going to learn the factors to consider when buying CBD oil.

Chapter Three: Factors To Consider When Buying CBD Oil

Given the numerous health benefits associated with CBD oil, you might be tempted to go out and buy the first CBD product you come across. Not so fast! The CBD marketplace is relatively new and because of this it is largely unregulated and lacks transparency. Some producers are taking advantage of the steadily rising popularity and the relative ignorance of customers to make a quick buck, all at the expense of users. Therefore, before you buy a CBD product, you need to take some time to do your homework and ensure that the product you are using is pure and safe for you to use. Don't be alarmed, below are some factors you need to watch out for when buying CBD products.

Product Quality

The hemp plant from which CBD is extracted is a bio-accumulator. This means that it absorbs elements and compounds that are present in the area in which the plant is grown, regardless of whether these elements and compounds are in the soil, the water, or even the air. This means that the conditions under which the hemp plant was grown affect the quality of the CBD extracted from it. If the hemp is grown using insecticides, pesticides, fertilizers, and other chemicals, it means that some traces of these chemicals will be present in the CBD taken from the plant.

Before purchasing a CBD product, you should research the seller and find out the conditions under which they grow their hemp. You should buy CBD products from sellers who extract their CBD from organic-certified hemp farms in pristine regions. This way, you can be certain that there are no impurities in their CBD products. You should also check whether the seller adds any other ingredients to their CBD products. Some products may contain solvents, preservatives, artificial coloring, sweeteners, and so on. Check these extra ingredients to ascertain that they are safe for you.

THC Levels

I mentioned earlier that CBD is typically extracted from hemp plants, which contains a very low concentration of the psychoactive compound THC. However, it is still possible that the extracted CBD might contain some traces of THC. Sometimes, some unscrupulous sellers might also extract their CBD from marijuana, which has a higher concentration of THC. In this case, the CBD might also contain a high percentage of THC. Before buying a CBD product, it is good to confirm whether it contains any THC.

Why do the THC levels matter? For some, having THC in their CBD product is not a big deal. However, it is important to note that using CBD oils with a high percentage of THC can lead to the THC showing up in drug tests. Therefore, if you work in an industry where you need to undergo drug tests, it might be wise to avoid CBD products that contain THC. It is also good to avoid

CBD products with a significant percentage of THC if you are going to be operating heavy machinery.

Legally, CBD products should have less than 0.3% of THC. This is what you should look for. Fortunately, many reputable sellers carry CBD products that have 0% THC. The question is, how do you know that the product has zero THC? This is where testing comes in. Before purchasing CBD products from a seller, you should confirm that the seller has a Certificate of Analysis (COA). The COA shows that the products being offered by the seller have been tested and shows all the details of the test. You should also confirm that the tests are recent.

CBD Concentration/Potency

Before buying CBD oil, you should also check the concentration or potency of the product. CBD oil does not contain CBD only. It will contain the carrier oil as well as other ingredients. Different CBD products will have varying amounts of CBD. For instance, one product might have 250mg of CBD per fluid ounce, while another product might have 1000mg of CBD per fluid ounce. The higher the concentration of CBD, the more potent the product, and stronger its effects. If you buy a CBD product with a very low concentration of CBD, the amount of CBD in the product might not even be enough to have any significant effect on your body. At the same time, buying a product with a very high CBD concentration might lead to very strong effects, especially if you are new to the use of CBD products.

Extraction Methods

The hemp plant contains hundreds of cannabinoids. Extracting these cannabinoids from the plant and separating CBD from the rest of the cannabinoids is a complicated process. There are several different methods of extracting CBD from hemp. The cheapest method of extracting CBD requires the use of harsh chemical solvents like butane, hexane, propane, isopropyl alcohol and ethanol to separate the CBD from the plant matter. Unfortunately, use of solvents often leaves a residue from these solvents in the CBB oil, leading to a lower quality CBD oil. The highest quality CBD is extracted using carbon dioxide. Carbon dioxide extraction does not leave any contaminants in the oil. Before purchasing a CBD product, you should confirm that the CBD was extracted using carbon dioxide instead of harsh solvents.

Price

When it comes to purchasing CBD products, don't always go for the cheapest product. I mentioned above that if you want high quality CBD products free of toxic contaminants, you should opt for CBD that was extracted using carbon dioxide. The carbon dioxide extraction process requires a high level expertise and complex equipment. As a result, it is not cheap. Therefore, CBD that has been extracted using carbon dioxide will generally be more expensive than CBD that has been extracted using other cheaper methods. Other factors that might contribute to CBD products being more expensive include the CBD being sourced from organically grown hemp, higher concentrations of CBD in the product and having the product subjected to testing. Therefore, if you notice that certain CBD products are a lot cheaper compared to other similar products, it might be wise to avoid them since the low price could be an indicator of low quality.

Full Spectrum vs. CBD Isolate

If you have already checked out some CBD products, you might have noticed that some are marketed as CBD "isolate" products while others are marketed as "full spectrum" CBD products. The difference between the two arises from their extraction methods. For CBD isolate products, the CBD is isolated from all the other cannabinoids that are found in the hemp plant. This means that the CBD is pure. Full spectrum products, on the other hand, do not separate the CBD from the other cannabinoids and terpenes found in the plant. So, which is better?

CBD isolate products are great for people who might be sensitive to one of the other compounds found in full spectrum products. Full spectrum CBD, on the other hand, is touted to be more effective than CBD isolate, because of something known as the "entourage effect". The entourage effect says that the sum effectiveness of all the cannabinoids working together is greater than the effectiveness of a single cannabinoid working in isolation. The concept of the entourage effect is supported by a study that was conducted by the Lautenberg Center for Immunology and Cancer Research, which found full spectrum CBD to be more effective than CBD isolate. While full spectrum CBD might be more effective, it is good to be cautious if you know you are going to be tested for drugs. Full spectrum contains trace amounts of THC, which can result in positive drug tests.

Natural vs. Synthetic CBD

In the first chapter, I mentioned that cannabinoids can be made naturally in the body, extracted from plants or made artificially in a lab. In a bid to increase their profit margins, some sellers might be selling CBD products made from synthetic CBD. I do not recommend this product. While synthetic CBD can be stronger than natural CBD, it often causes negative side effects, such as confusion, vomiting, and rapid heartbeat. Therefore, you should avoid CBD products made from synthetic CBD.

Watch Out For Fake Sellers

With the rising popularity and demand for CBD products, it is inevitable that there will be some scammers trying to cash in on the trend, especially for those buying their CBD products online. There are ways to be careful before making a purchase. Watch out for sellers who use excessive sales techniques, like greatly exaggerating the benefits of CBD oil. Before making a purchase, it is good to check online reviews to find out what other customers are saying about the seller. If you buy from fake sellers, you might end up with low quality and ineffective products.

Despite the growing popularity of the use of CBD oil and the numerous health benefits associated with CBD products, don't rush in to your purchase. Take time to do your research and evaluate the seller and their product. By the time you decide to buy, you should be sure that the product you are buying is safe for you and that it will give you whatever health benefit you are searching for.

Chapter Summary

- You should take the time to do some research about the CBD product and the seller before you make a purchase.
- The first thing you need to check for is the quality of the product. Ensure the CBD product you are buying does not contain any chemicals or impurities.
- You should also check for THC levels in the CBD oil and check for a COA (Certificate of Analysis) to ascertain that the THC levels and other details listed on the product are correct.
- You should check the potency of the CBD oil. Low potency products might not be effective.
- Opt for CBD products that use the carbon dioxide extraction method, since it results in higher quality CBD that is free from impurities.
- Be wary of very cheap CBD products. The extremely low price might be an indicator of low quality.
- Check whether the CBD product is full spectrum or a CBD isolate. While full spectrum products might

be more effective, they may trigger positive drug tests since they contain THC.

- ☐ Avoid buying products made from synthetic CBD, which often lead to negative side effects.
- ☐ Finally, you should watch out for fake sellers and scammers who might end up selling you low quality, ineffective products.

In the next chapter, you are going to learn how to use CBD oil.

Chapter Four: How To Use CBD Oil For First Timers

If it is your first time using CBD oil, the process can be a bit confusing. Deciding the best way to use CBD oil, as well as the correct dosages required for you, is important. There are five major methods of delivering CBD into your system. The best method for you will depend on your lifestyle and what you want to achieve by incorporating CBD oil into your lifestyle.

The five delivery methods for CBD are as follows:

1. Inhalation
2. Topical Application
3. Sublingual Delivery
4. Ingestion
5. Transdermal Delivery

Inhalation

Inhalation is the fastest and the most efficient way of delivering CBD into your system. Inhalation also allows the most CBD to get absorbed into the bloodstream compared to other methods. When you take CBD oil through inhalation, it goes into the alveoli in your lungs and from there it is directly absorbed into your blood. Due to the speedy absorption, inhalation is the best method for those looking for a quick remedy. People taking CBD oil to help ease pain or anxiety should consider inhalation, since the effects will be felt almost immediately. CBD delivered to the body through inhalation also passes out of the bloodstream much faster compared to other delivery methods.

For those who prefer to deliver CBD into the body through inhalation, the CBD oil comes in the form of vaporizer e-juice that you can use with a vape pen. Alternatively, you can use the CBD oil e-juice on a desktop vaporizer.

Despite its speed and effectiveness, inhalation is recommended for people with some vaping experience. It is not recommended for children because it can be a bit complicated to teach a child how to use vape pens. Additionally, using this method can make it difficult to accurately control the dosage of CBD going into the body.

Topical Application

In chapter one, I mentioned that cannabinoid receptors are located all over the body, including inside organs like the skin. This means that CBD can be absorbed into the body through the skin. There are several products that are meant to be applied directly on the skin. These come in the form of lotions, creams, salves, moisturizers, soaps and shampoos. Unlike other delivery methods, topical application does not get CBD into the bloodstream. Instead, the CBD only works on the area of the skin where it has been applied. This makes topical application a good method for relieving pain and inflammation. You only need to rub the CBD oil directly on joints, sore muscles, or other places that might be experiencing some pain.

Since topical application does not get the CBD into your bloodstream, it is considered a lot safer than other methods, since you don't have to worry about excessive dosage or frequent use. Unlike inhalation, topical application is a bit slow. It might take up to an hour before you start feeling the effects of the CBD oil. If you want the effects to last longer, you might need to keep applying the CBD oil to the affected area every couple of hours. CBD products meant to be applied topically may also need a high concentration of CBD to be effective, which means they are more likely to be expensive.

Sublingual Delivery

This method involves delivering CBD directly into the bloodstream through the capillaries found in the mucous membrane inside the mouth. With this method, the CBD oil is administered in the form of liquid concentrate drops known as tinctures. Tinctures are made by mixing highly concentrated liquid CBD extracts with a solvent liquid base, such as vegetable glycerin or apple cider vinegar.

With this method, the tinctures or droplets of CBD oil are dropped under the tongue. The droplets are held under the tongue for up to two minutes, allowing the mucous membrane of the mouth to absorb the CBD. After the two minutes are over, any remaining CBD that has not been absorbed can be swallowed and allowed to get into the system through digestion.

Sublingual application is the second quickest method of delivering CBD into your system. The CBD is absorbed directly into the bloodstream, bypassing the digestive system and the liver. With sublingual delivery, the effects of the CBD can be felt within a few minutes. The effects also last much longer compared to inhalation. Do not place the CBD oil droplets on your tongue since you are more likely to swallow the droplets and send them to the digestive system where absorption is much slower

Ingestion

This is the simplest method of delivering CBD into the body, which makes it a good option for children and beginners. No training is required with this method since all you need to do is swallow the edible and you are good to go. When CBD oil is delivered to the body through ingestion, it goes through the digestive system and the liver. The CBD is absorbed into your bloodstream through the liver in the same way most vitamins are absorbed into the body. Since the CBD has to pass through the digestive system and the liver, this method is not particularly fast. It might take anywhere between thirty minutes to an hour before you start feeling the effects of the CBD. In addition, the edibles in which the CBD is contained as well as any other foods you eat might affect how the CBD is absorbed into the body, minimizing its effects.

CBD oil meant for ingestion can be mixed with a variety of food products. It comes in the form of juices, candies, capsules, baked goods, beverages, salad dressings, and so on. You can also buy the CBD oil and use it at home when cooking your meals.

Transdermal Delivery

Finally, CBD can be delivered into the body through transdermal patches. The transdermal CBD patch is placed into the body just like birth control patches and nicotine patches. The patch then gradually releases CBD into the body where it is absorbed through the skin and the surrounding capillaries. Transdermal delivery of CBD is fairly easy and quite convenient. Since the CBD is constantly and gradually released into the body, the effects of the CBD are long lasting. Since the CBD is released in predetermined amounts, the dosage can be controlled accurately when using this method.

What's The Best Dosage?

Apart from the choice of delivery method, the thing that new users of CBD oil find confusing is how to determine the best dosage. Since the use of CBD oil as a supplement started relatively recently, the FDA has not come up with a Recommended Daily Intake like it has for other supplements. In other words, there is no official dosage for CBD. This can make it quite confusing for users to determine how much CBD they need to take. One of the most common dosage recommendations is that a person should take a dropper per day. However, even this is not an accurate way of determining the right dosage. This is because it does not take into account a number of factors that can affect the dosage, such as the concentration of CBD in the product, the weight, tolerance, genetics and general health of the individual, the body chemistry of the individual, and the severity of condition the person is trying to treat.

To make matters even more confusing, an individual's body physiology is not static. It keeps changing. As it changes, the endocannabinoid system and the cannabinoid receptors, which interact with CBD, change with it. Therefore, a dosage that worked today might not work a year down the line. So, with all these variables, how do you determine the best dosage for you? While there are no hard and fast rules, there are three general guidelines to follow to determine the optimal dosage for you. These are:

☐ **Your Body Weight:**
  ○ Like with most supplements, your body weight has an impact on the effectiveness of the supplement. Generally, the heavier you weigh,

the more CBD you will require. A good guideline for determining the right dosage based on your weight is for every 10 pounds of body weight, you should take 1-6 mg of CBD, depending on the intensity of the pain you are experiencing.

- **Start Small And Increase Gradually:**
  - Even when two people have a similar body weight, taking similar doses of CBD will not always lead to the same effects. Therefore, you need to adjust your dosage to achieve the best results based on your body. After determining your initial dosage based on your weight, you should take that dosage and observe how it affects your body. If it does not achieve the desired effects, you can gradually increase the dosage while continuing to observe your body until you find the optimal dosage for your condition. This trial and error method is very important to keep in mind.
- **Talk To Your Physician**

- If you are unsure of how much CBD you should take, it is wise to seek the advice of a physician, especially if you are using CBD to treat a serious medical condition. The physician can help you determine the best dosage based on the intensity of your condition and your body's reaction to CBD.

- As I close this chapter, I want you to understand one thing. While the use of CBD oil has been approved by the World Health Organization as safe for almost everyone, it might cause some unexpected reactions, especially if you are on medication or if you are pregnant. If you have some concerns about how CBD oil might react with any medications you are taking, or if you are unsure whether CBD oil is safe for you because of your condition, you should speak with your physician before you start using any CBD product.

Chapter Summary

- [ ] There are five major methods of delivering CBD into your system.
- [ ] Inhalation is the fastest and the most efficient way of delivering CBD into your system, though it is difficult to accurately control the dosage of CBD going into the body.
- [ ] Applying CBD oil on the skin is a good option for relieving pain and inflammation, thought it takes some time for the effect to be felt.
- [ ] Sublingual application is the second quickest method of delivering CBD into your system. The effects are fast and last much longer than other methods.
- [ ] Ingestion is the simplest method of delivering CBD into the body, which makes it a good option for children and beginners. However, it is a bit slow and might be affected by accompanying foodstuffs.
- [ ] Transdermal delivery of CBD is easy and convenient, and allows for accurate control of your dosage. Its effects are also quite long lasting.

- There is no officially recommended dosage for CBD. The optimum dosage varies from person to person.
- The three general guidelines you should follow to determine the optimal dosage for you is to use your body weight, start small and increase gradually, and consult a physician whenever you are in doubt.

In the next chapter, we are going to look at some success stories from people who are already using CBD oil.

Chapter Five: Success Stories Of People Using CBD Oil

In the last few years, owing to the media hype around the numerous health benefits of CBD oil and confirmation of these benefits by a growing body of research, more and more people have successfully incorporated CBD oil into their lives. In this chapter, we are going to take a look at the stories of people who have experienced positive results after using CBD oil products.

CBD Oil Helped Juan Deal With Sleep Issues

Juan had been having sleep problems for a while. On most nights, sleep did not come easily. He would spend more than an hour in bed trying to fall asleep. Other times, he found himself waking up in the middle of the night. He would remain in bed for long periods of time - tossing and turning - failing to fall back asleep. His sleep issues had even started causing problems at his workplace. Due to his lack of sleep, Juan became moody and highly irritable. He would shout and snap at colleagues for the flimsiest reasons. His productivity at work also started taking a dip. He tried a number of conventional methods of dealing with sleep issues but for some reason they were not helping.

When sharing his woes with a friend, a CBD aficionado himself, suggested that Juan should try using CBD oil to treat his problem. Juan was skeptical, but he was willing to try anything to help him sleep. He started taking a few drops of CBD oil every evening before going to bed. Within a few days, there was a great improvement in Juan's sleep quality. It became easier for him to fall asleep. He also stopped waking up in the middle of the night. Due to the increased quality and quantity of sleep, his productivity at work improved and he stopped being moody. To this day, Juan continues using CBD oil, not only for the sleeping problems, but for other health problems as well.

CBD Oil Helped Marissa Quit Smoking

Marissa had been smoking for about five years. After seeing a close relative suffer from lung cancer as a result of smoking, Marissa decided it was time for her to quit. Unfortunately, if you have been smoking for five years, it's not that easy. She tried various methods of quitting but she just could not make any stick. Each time she tried, she always found herself going back for one last cigarette, which would be followed by many more. During a group therapy session, someone mentioned that he had successfully used CBD oil to deal with his smoking addiction, and Marissa decided to give it a try.

Marissa started taking CBD every morning after waking up. She found that instead of craving a cigarette in the morning, her cravings came much later in the day. She went from five cigarettes a day to two cigarettes. She added another dose of CBD after lunch, which helped her reduce her smoking to one cigarette a day. Finally, she was able to completely do away with smoking. At the time of this writing it has been a year since Marissa smoked her last cigarette, and she is grateful for having discovered CBD oil. Without it, she doubts that she would have been able to quit smoking.

CBD Oil Helped Brittany's Daughter Deal With Seizures

When Brittany gave birth to a baby girl, she was ecstatic. She was so happy to be a mother. Unfortunately, her joy was short lived. Once her daughter was five months old, she started experiencing seizures. Brittany took her daughter to several hospitals but nothing seemed to work. Her daughter was given multiple medications, including Klonopin and Depakote, but they did not stop her seizures. These medications also came with terrible side effects. It seemed they were only making things worse for Brittany's daughter.

Brittany was desperate to try anything that would help her daughter, and when she heard about CBD therapy, she didn't have any second thoughts about trying it. However, there was one problem. She was told that CBD oil is most effective when it contains some THC as well. Unfortunately, her state did not allow the sale and use of any products containing THC. Brittany decided to move to Colorado, where state laws allow the sale of products containing THC. Brittany's daughter was put on CBD therapy using CBD oil that also contained higher levels of THC (above the 0.3% recommended by other states). This turned out to be a life saver for her daughter. After she started her CBD therapy, the daughter's seizures have reduced by more than 90%. In addition, CBD therapy does not cause any negative side effects, unlike the prescription medications she had used at first.

CBD Oil Cured Her Dad's Tumor

In April 2017, Danielle's dad started complaining of abdominal pains. When he went to the hospital for a check-up, it was discovered that he had a bile duct carcinoma. The carcinoma was in advanced stages. The doctors declared that he would not live for more than one year. Danielle and her dad were devastated. A few weeks after the diagnosis, he started suffering from jaundice and got admitted into a hospital. After doing some research, Danielle and her family decided to transfer her father to a different hospital where CBD oil was included in his treatment.

After he started taking CBD oil, his condition started improving. After about two weeks, he was discharged but continued going to the hospital for routine check-ups. About six months after he started the CBD treatment, scan results showed no signs of a tumor in his bile ducts. He is completely healed. It has been more than a year since the doctors claimed that he had less than one year to live, and he is now completely healthy and normal.

CBD Oil Helped Charlotte Deal With Dravet Syndrome

Charlotte's case is perhaps one of the most famous success stories of CBD oil and how it can improve a person's quality of life. Charlotte Figi was born a healthy child alongside her fraternal twin sister. Three months after her birth, however, Charlotte experienced her first epileptic seizure. This was followed by another seizure a week later. By the time she was two years old, the frequency of the seizures had greatly increased, with seizures occurring daily. Despite numerous tests, doctors did not find anything wrong with her. When she was two and a half years old, she was taken to the Children's Hospital in Colorado, where she was diagnosed with Dravet Syndrome.

Now, here is the thing with Dravet Syndrome. It has no cure. Children suffering from this condition do not typically survive beyond early childhood. Knowing the clock was ticking away on their daughter's life, Charlotte's parents were eager to try anything, from keto diets to experimental drugs used to reduce seizures in dogs. By the time she was six years old, the seizures became too much. She was experiencing up to 300 seizures a week. The seizures affected her ability to eat, talk, and even walk. Even her cognitive development started lagging behind her twin sister's. It was at this time that Charlotte's father stumbled upon a video of a boy who used a CBD treatment to cure a similar condition.

Out of desperation, Charlotte's parents decided to try out CBD. After she started the CBD treatment, Charlotte's seizures stopped almost immediately. After her first dosage, she went several days without experiencing a seizure, which was a huge relief for her and her parents, considering she had typically experienced several seizures each day. With the help of CBD oil, Charlotte's life was turned around and she was able to live like a normal child. Her case was so remarkable that the strain of cannabis from which she got her CBD oil was named Charlotte's Web in her honor. Today, Charlotte's Web has become one of the most effective treatments for children suffering from Dravet Syndrome.

CBD Oil Helped Shannon Deal With Anxiety And Depression

Shannon was one of the 40 million adults in America suffering from anxiety disorders and depression. Shannon experienced extreme anxiety and panic attacks every time she left the house. Her extreme anxiety affected both her personal and professional life. She even experienced a suicidal episode and once attempted to take her life.

Seeing the suffering she was going through, her psychiatrist suggested that she try out CBD pills. After she started using the CBD pills, Shannon experienced a tremendous change. Her panic attacks stopped completely. Today, she does not have any issues with anxiety and depression, and she uses CBD as a regular supplement.

This is only a handful of stories from people who have successfully used CBD oil. There are numerous others who have used CBD oil to successfully deal with various health and wellness issues. However, these six stories are a sampling that show CBD oil can have a profound impact on the quality of your life.

Chapter Summary

- Juan used CBD oil to deal with his sleep issues. From finding it hard to fall asleep to waking up in the middle of the night, CBD oil made it easier for Juan to fall asleep and ended his midnight insomnia.

- Having tried different methods to quit smoking to no avail, Marissa was finally able to successfully quit smoking by using CBD oil.

- CBD oil helped Brittany reduce her daughter's seizures by more than 90% without any negative side effects.

- CBD oil cured Danielle's dad, who had a tumor in his bile duct, and gave him another chance at life despite doctors having claimed he had less than a year to live.

- CBD oil gave Charlotte a chance at a normal childhood. She went from 300 seizures a week to about one or two seizures a month.

- Shannon used CBD oil to successfully deal with anxiety and depression.

In the next chapter, you are going to learn about some common myths and misconceptions about CBD oil.

Chapter Six: Common Myths And Misconceptions About CBD Oil

The numerous health benefits associated with CBD oil have created a lot of interest in it. In a bid to make it even more popular and push its adoption, over-zealous aficionados and the sensationalist media have created a lot of hype and buzz around CBD products. Unfortunately, some of the information making the rounds is not true. If you are not familiar with the topic of CBD oil, you might find yourself falling prey to misinformation about CBD. In this chapter we take a look at some common myths and misconceptions about CBD oil. This will make it easier for you to tell apart fact from fiction. Below are the seven most common myths.

Myth 1: Hemp And Marijuana Are The Same

People often use the terms hemp, marijuana, and cannabis interchangeably. When they hear that CBD is extracted from hemp, they wrongly assume that it is extracted from marijuana. There is a difference between the two. The confusion stems from the fact that the word cannabis is an umbrella term for the two plants. Cannabis is a species of plants that contain cannabinoids. Hemp and marijuana are two subspecies within the cannabis sativa species. The difference between the two plants is a result of their THC concentrations. Hemp has very low concentrations of THC (less than 0.3%) and marijuana can contain as much as 12% THC. Because of its high THC content, marijuana is not typically used for the production of CBD oil, even though it contains CBD. Marijuana is primarily used for medical and recreational purposes but hemp is used in the production of CBD oil, ropes, and plastics.

Myth 2: CBD Oil Can Get You High

When people hear the term cannabis, they automatically associate it with weed and getting high. When people hear that CBD oil comes from cannabis, they assume that it can get you high. However, CBD is not psychoactive, therefore it cannot get you high. THC is the cannabinoid that is responsible for the feelings of highness. For CBD oils to be sold legally in most states, it needs to have less than 0.3% THC, which is not nearly enough to produce psychoactive effects. Also, using most CBD oil products will not result in positive drug tests. Drug tests check for THC, not CBD. Therefore, you don't have to worry about triggering a positive drug test after using CBD oil products. However, you should make sure that the CBD oil products you are using have less than 0.3% THC. If you buy products with a high quantity of THC, it will show on your drug test.

Myth 3: CBD Is Medical While THC Is Recreational

Many people assume that CBD is the medically useful part of the cannabis plant while THC is only useful for recreation. This is not entirely true. Despite its psychoactive properties THC also has some great therapeutic properties. Just like CBD, THC has great anti-inflammatory properties. It is also great for boosting your appetite. In fact, multiple studies show that CBD is most effective when it is coupled with some THC. The two cannabinoids enhance each other's therapeutic effects when they work together. One study conducted by researchers from the California Pacific Medical Center found that CBD is more potent against tumors when it is combined with THC. CBD's anti-inflammatory effects are also more potent when it is combined with THC.

Myth 4: High Doses Of CBD Are More Effective Than Low Doses

People wrongfully assume that when it comes to CBD, more is better. This is not always true. Sometimes, low doses might actually be more effective than high doses. This is because CBD is biphasic. This means that low amounts of CBD can produce effects that are totally opposite to the effects of high amounts. For instance, low doses of CBD will give you a mild burst of energy, whereas a higher dose will promote sleep. Therefore, your dose should be determined by the condition you are trying to treat. Do not assume that a higher dose will always be more effective in dealing with each and every condition.

Myth 5: CBD Turns Into THC Once It Gets Into The Body

This is the most outrageous misconception I have heard about CBD. While it is not clear where this myth originated, it has been spread a lot in online forums and even claims to be backed by scientific tests. However, this myth is just that – a myth. There is no scientific evidence that the body converts CBD into THC.

Myth 6: CBD Hemp Oil Is The Same As Hemp Seed Oil

Some unscrupulous sellers might take advantage of this myth to pass off hemp seed oil as CBD hemp oil. While both products come from the same plant, hemp seed oil does not contain CBD. Hemp seed oil comes from a part of the plant that has no CBD, namely, the seeds of the hemp plant. CBD hemp oil, on the other hand, is extracted from the leaves and flowers, which are rich in CBD. While hemp seed oil also has several nutritional benefits, it does not have the health benefits of CBD oil. You should watch out to make sure you are not purchasing hemp seed oil instead of CBD hemp oil.

Myth 7: CBD Oil Is Not Safe For Children

Many people assume that CBD oil is not safe for children and will avoid using it on children unless there is no other option. However, CBD oil can be used safely by people of all ages. Several studies conducted by researchers from various universities in the United States indicate that CBD does not have any negative effects on children. Another study conducted by Dr. Leslie Iversen from Oxford University found that CBD and other cannabinoids are actually safer than aspirin.

Chapter Summary

- People often use the terms marijuana and hemp interchangeably. However, marijuana is THC rich while hemp is CBD rich. CBD products are typically extracted from hemp, not marijuana.

- People wrongly assume that CBD oil products can get you high and show up in drug tests. However, CBD products will not get you high or show up in drug tests provided they have less than 0.3% THC.

- Many people assume that CBD is the medically useful part of the cannabis plant while THC is only useful for recreation. Both cannabinoids have therapeutic effects and may actually be more effective when working together.

- People wrongfully assume that when it comes to CBD, more is better. However, low doses might sometimes be more effective than high doses.

- Some people claim that CBD turns into THC inside the body. This is simply not true.

- People often think that all hemp products are the same. However, hemp seed oil is different from CBD hemp oil since it does not contain any CBD.
- Some people think CBD oil is not safe for children. However, research shows that CBD oil can be used safely by people of all ages.

Final Words

Thank you for sticking with me to the end of this book.

By now, you know all the basics you need to know about CBD oil products and how they can help you improve the quality of your life. You know where CBD comes from and why it does not get you high like other cannabis products. You are aware of the numerous health benefits of CBD oil, the things to be wary of when buying CBD products, and how to use CBD oil products if you are just getting started. You have read the real-life stories of people who have successfully used CBD products in their lives - you know that the benefits of CBD oil are not just mere claims. You also know of the misconceptions associated with CBD oil, therefore you are in a much better position to know when someone tries to dupe you.

Armed with this information, you have all you need to start incorporating CBD oil into your lifestyle and reap the health benefits that it comes with.

Cheers to a healthier and better life!

Did You Like This Book?

If you enjoyed this book, I would like to ask you for a favor. Would you be kind enough to share your thoughts and post a review of this book? Just a few sentences would already be really helpful.

Your voice is important for this book to reach as many people as possible.

The more reviews this book gets, the more people will be able to find it and also learn about the wonderful health benefits of CBD hemp oil.

***

IF YOU DID NOT LIKE THIS BOOK, THEN PLEASE TELL ME!

You can email me at **feedback@semsoli.com**, to share with me what you did not like.

Perhaps I can change it.

A book does not have to be stagnant, in today's world. With feedback from readers like yourself, I can improve the book. So, you can impact the quality of this book, and I welcome your feedback. Help make this book better for everyone!

Thank you again for reading this book and good luck with applying everything you have learned!

I'm rooting for you...

Notes

www.ingramcontent.com/pod-product-compliance
Lightning Source LLC
Chambersburg PA
CBHW071244020426
42333CB00015B/1627